AUTUMN WYNTERS

Health Benefits of Crocheting
Endless Reasons to Love It - A Craft or Creative Hobby Is Not All It Is

Copyright © 2022 by Autumn Wynters

All rights reserved. No part of this publication may be reproduced, stored or transmitted in any form or by any means, electronic, mechanical, photocopying, recording, scanning, or otherwise without written permission from the publisher. It is illegal to copy this book, post it to a website, or distribute it by any other means without permission.

Autumn Wynters asserts the moral right to be identified as the author of this work.

Autumn Wynters has no responsibility for the persistence or accuracy of URLs for external or third-party Internet Websites referred to in this publication and does not guarantee that any content on such Websites is, or will remain, accurate or appropriate.

Designations used by companies to distinguish their products are often claimed as trademarks. All brand names and product names used in this book and on its cover are trade names, service marks, trademarks and registered trademarks of their respective owners. The publishers and the book are not associated with any product or vendor mentioned in this book. None of the companies referenced within the book have endorsed the book.

First edition

This book was professionally typeset on Reedsy.
Find out more at reedsy.com

Contents

1	INTRODUCTION	1
2	WHY CROCHETING SHOULD BE YOUR NEW HOBBY	4
3	WHY ALL THE CRAZE ABOUT CROCHETING?	6
4	GETTING STARTED	8
5	THE CREATIVE POTENTIAL OF CROCHET	11
6	THE ART OF CROCHET IS SUITABLE FOR ALL AGES	13
7	HEALTH BENEFITS OF CROCHETING	15
8	THE SECRET TO A 20-MINUTE SOLUTION	23
9	CROCHET ENCOURAGES SOCIAL CONNECTION BY COMBATING LONELINESS	24
10	CROCHET PROVIDES ENDLESS GIFT POSSIBILITIES!	28
11	CROCHET HAS INCOME-EARNING POTENTIAL	30
12	DONATIONS CAN BE MADE TO HOSPITALS OR TO THOSE IN NEED	32
13	15 AWESOME RESOURCES FOR BEGINNERS	34
14	CONCLUSION	39
15	RESOURCES	41

1

INTRODUCTION

WELCOME As one gets older you realize that it takes practice and patience to learn a new skill and it is not something you can just pick up overnight. I allowed myself to be more forgiving of mistakes and learn something the wrong way, and it also teaches you how to make it right and not repeat the same mistakes. You learn how to problem solve and can even find a different solution to the original problem.

During my freshman year of college, I was stressed out during finals week. Instead of reading books, I decided to search YouTube for stress-relieving hobbies. One of the videos just so happened to be a group of crocheters who were making beautiful works of lovely art and teaching step-by-step how-to videos online. In comparison to reading or staring at pictures or words in a book, the videos were more captivating. My learning style has changed since I realized this. My project would never look right at the end no matter how much I read and stared at pictures. It became apparent to me that audio and visual learning was more effective for me.

I definitely discovered my learning style through crocheting. The most exciting part of the experience was watching how each stitch was created step by step and seeing my own creations come to life. I developed my crocheting skills by rewinding, watching again, and listening again and again. When you're learning a new skill, having a completed project at the end of every video is a great confidence booster.

The process was easy this time, and I found it to be both relaxing and fun. Studying for my finals, quizzes, projects, papers, essays, and all the reading necessary to graduate in college with a BSN in nursing requires a great deal of time. My crocheting helped me keep calm, relieve stress, and deal with anxiety while I was in college. The stitch was easier this "millionth time" around - start with a slip knot, add a row of chain stitches, then use a cluster of three double crochet stitches with wide spaces in between clusters - and I could see exactly where each stitch should go as I worked on the blanket. I counted the clusters and even edges the whole way up. It was a great experience, and I actually had time to make a project (and a whole blanket, no less!)

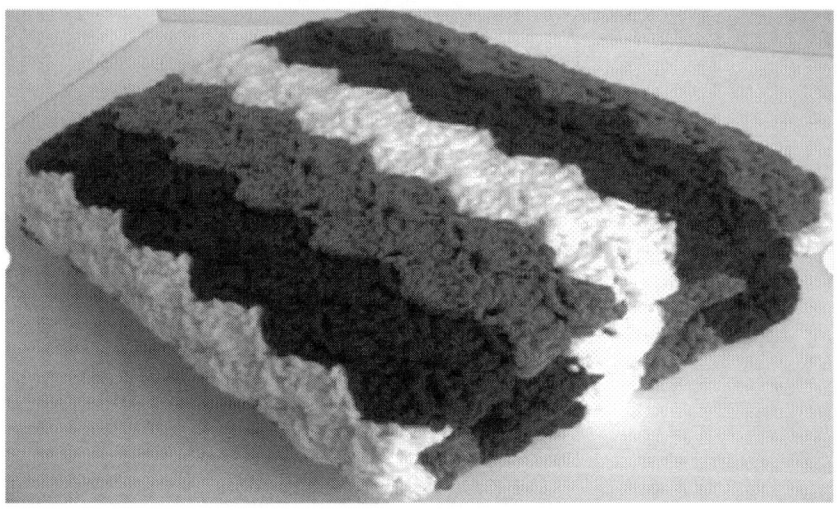

INTRODUCTION

In addition to that first cluster pattern (called a granny stripe if you're interested), I have crocheted dozens of afghans using increasingly more complex stitches and patterns. It's always a delight to give handmade items of love as gifts to friends and family on special occasions. Over the years, I've designed and made shawls, hats, mittens, scarves, socks, amigurumi and doll clothes, necklaces, and dollhouse furniture. Crochet is one of the mad skills that I have no end to. I love it!

2

WHY CROCHETING SHOULD BE YOUR NEW HOBBY

THE IMPACT
Crocheting garments by hand is a way to improve the environment and improve the quality of life for everyone.

By doing so, you protect the maker's rights and ensure a fair working environment, as well as ensuring that many yarns in use today are ethically sourced and responsibly produced. Additionally, recycled and upcycled yarns have emerged as a relatively new trend in the textile industry, but one that is expected to continue to grow.

Moreover, crochet offers many opportunities for connecting with other makers. There is something magical about being part of a crafter's community, whether you participate in a local sip-and-stitch group or interact with other crafters on social media.

Personally, the quiet repetition of crochet reduces stress (aka a lifesaver for mothers of young children). Is there a better reason to jump on the crochet bandwagon than that? The next time someone asks you "Where did you get that cute sweater?" You can simply reply, "I made it!

WHY CROCHETING SHOULD BE YOUR NEW HOBBY

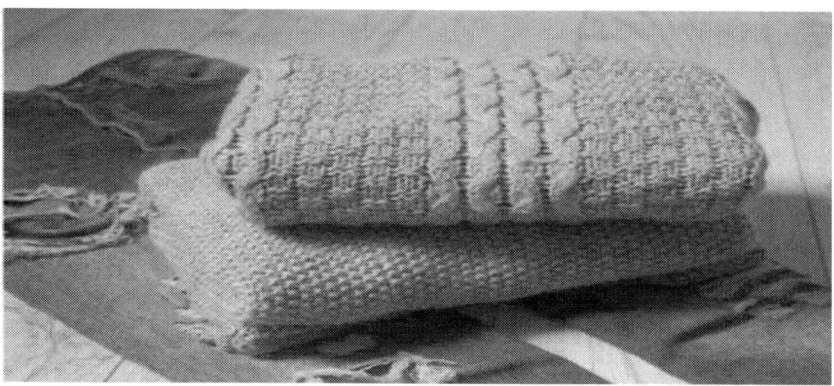

Here's the surprise!

You can crochet a blanket in no time at all. It is very easy to learn basic crochet stitches by watching a YouTube video, and you only need a crochet hook and acrylic yarn to get started.

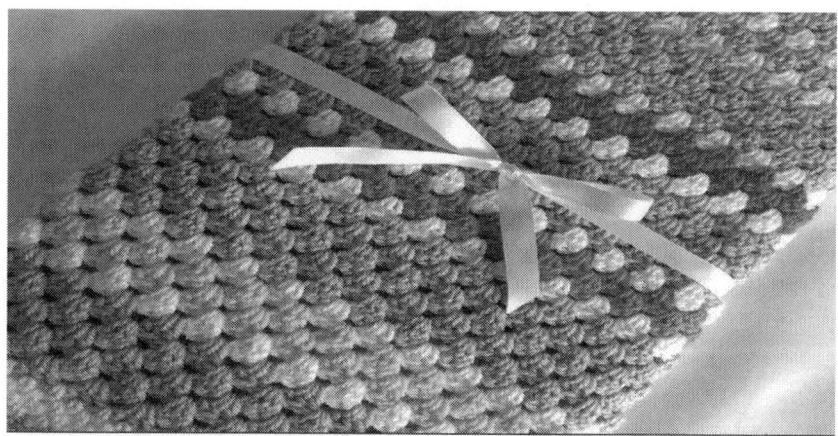

You can take advantage of crochet to improve your health. You can learn to crochet for numerous reasons, including real benefits that have been proven by science. As an activity that promotes healing and relieves stress, crochet is more than just a craft you do for fun. You may find crochet to be the answer to your prayers when you learn why and how it may be beneficial.

3

WHY ALL THE CRAZE ABOUT CROCHETING?

Learning to crochet can be started with only a few small purchases, such as acrylic or cotton yarn, which are both fairly cheap. Crocheting and other yarn crafts are gaining popularity for a variety of reasons, including social media attention on Instagram. It's pretty awesome that crochet entrepreneurs and those interested in learning the craft can connect and showcase their projects. Crocheting's popularity isn't exclusively due to that reason, however.

If I'm being bold here, I think the primary reason for the renewed interest in crocheting can be attributed to the need for a sense of purpose during uncertain times. People have been forced to change their lives dramatically over the past two and a half years.

It might have been necessary to work from home, be laid off, or resign in order to provide childcare and schoolwork assistance. COVID-19 caused a significant upheaval in a world where most people are accustomed to the routine, which left many people feeling lost in stressful waters. There's something very relaxing about crocheting because it's monotonous: you do the same stitch over and over until you almost don't see it anymore. It gives you time to let your mind wander and just be without having to concentrate.

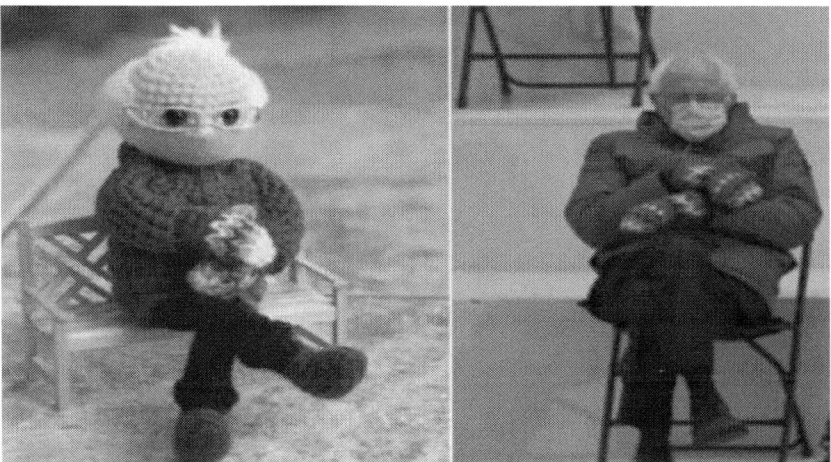

A growing number of people are discovering that crocheting is wonderful for their minds, bodies, and spirits. We have endless reasons to convince you to pick up a crochet hook if you've been debating whether or not to do so. Just be aware that you might find yourself in the middle of an impulse trip to the craft store as a result.

4

GETTING STARTED

CROCHETING IS INEXPENSIVE

You Can Learn To Crochet Too! The cost of starting some hobbies can be prohibitive. This is not the case with crochet. The cost of learning to crochet is extremely reasonable, and you only need a few items in order to get started. A crochet hook, colored yarn (I recommend a yarn weight of 4/worsted weight yarn for beginners), and scissors are all it takes to get started. A crochet hook with an ergonomic handle is no more expensive than a regular one but is much more comfortable to use.

It really only takes one hook to get started. It's important to check the yarn label for the correct hook size if you're going to buy just one hook. The more experienced you become, the more advanced your projects can be, using different hook sizes, stitches, and yarns. There are also a lot of cheap yarns available. You'll find skeins at craft stores or online, and if you look around, you can always find them on sale.

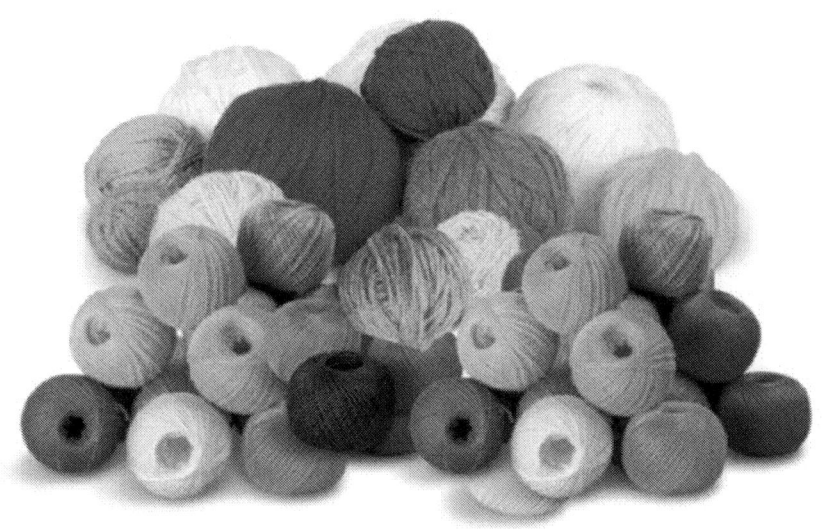

There are also hundreds of free tutorial videos and online resources available if you have never attempted crochet before. Free crochet patterns can be found on many websites, from those for beginners to those for advanced crocheters.

When learning to follow patterns, you should have a variety of hooks on hand. Getting a set that has multiple sizes is definitely possible without busting your budget. Below is a link to a reasonably priced Crochet Kit on Amazon: **https://a.co/d/ePlyJHn**

HEALTH BENEFITS OF CROCHETING

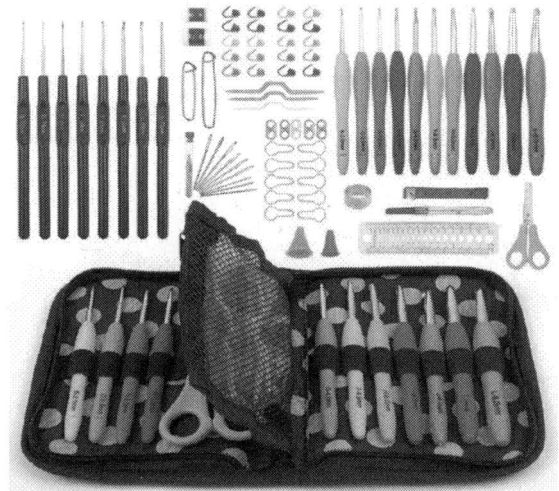

The best thing you can do when you are just starting out is to buy inexpensive yarn. It's perfect for practicing. In time, you may be able to graduate to more expensive yarns as you become more proficient at the craft. Overall, you can get everything you need to get started crocheting for around ten or fifteen dollars. **Now isn't that pretty reasonable?**

5

THE CREATIVE POTENTIAL OF CROCHET

No matter what your passion is, you can find a crochet project that showcases your creativity and talent. Is your favorite literary character a character you would like to crochet miniatures of? If you like Anne of Green Gables, there's a crochet kit for you (hello!). Is crocheting your own swimsuit on your bucket list? You have nothing to fear, oh progressive swimmer. Those, too, have patterns. Whether you design your own innovative crochet patterns or incorporate your favorite colors into infinity scarves, the creative possibilities are limitless.

A crocheter's skills can always be improved. One of the reasons why crocheting appeals to me is that I am very goal-oriented. It's easy to start by learning basic stitches and starting smaller projects, and even those early attempts can be improved and perfected as you learn.

HEALTH BENEFITS OF CROCHETING

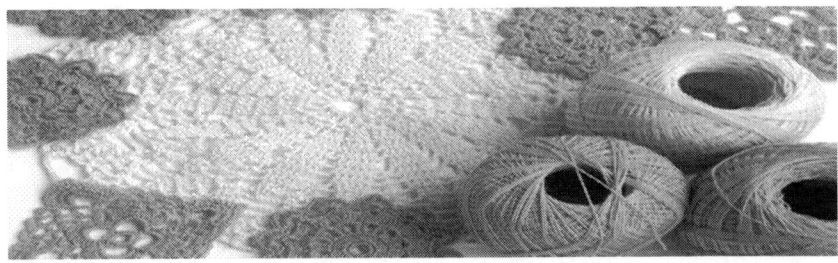

You can also challenge yourself to more elaborate stitching techniques and advanced patterns once you've mastered the basics of crochet. When you take up crocheting as a hobby, you are always on the lookout for something new to learn, which later increases your self-esteem and confidence.

6

THE ART OF CROCHET IS SUITABLE FOR ALL AGES

It is not possible to teach crochet to a toddler, but children as young as five can begin learning the basics. From there, you can introduce very simple patterns once they have gained comfort crocheting on their own. That's one of the things I love about crocheting - there's no minimum level of experience required to learn this crafty skill. Many people can find something appealing in the crochet world, from teenagers to grandmas.

HEALTH BENEFITS OF CROCHETING

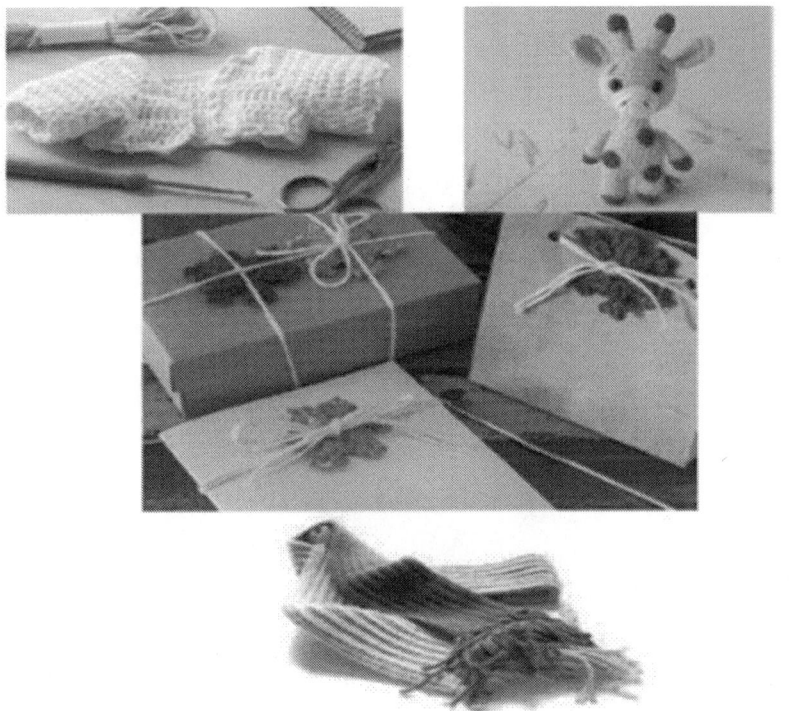

Crochet is actually one of the easiest crafts to learn out of all the new crafts you could learn. Compared to knitting, I find it much easier. It also gives you a wider range of options. In addition, it allows you to be more adaptable.

7

HEALTH BENEFITS OF CROCHETING

A　**NXIETY AND DEPRESSION CAN BE MANAGED WITH CROCHET**
Millions of individuals are struggling to manage anxiety and despair. According to the Center for Infectious Disease Research and Policy, depression rates increased under COVID-19, and it's easy to see how the social and physical constraints imposed may have a detrimental influence.

Numerous benefits can be gained from crocheting for those suffering from anxiety and depression. While crocheting, you can concentrate on the task at hand instead of the many thoughts circling in your head. You can also relax and return to the present moment by crocheting with colors that are relaxing and soothing.

CONFIDENCE IS BUILT THROUGH CROCHET
The feeling of accomplishment you may have experienced when you finally mastered a new skill may be empowering if you have ever struggled to master one. It's always a joy to see my godson's and goddaughter's faces light up when something they've worked hard to make comes out delicious. In addition to boosting your self-esteem, crochet is also a powerful confidence booster when you learn a variety

of techniques and use them to make stunning pieces.

As you gain experience, it will become easier to hear someone else admire your work. To get the ball rolling, you need to learn only a few stitches. Even if you only learn how to make a chain and single crochet, you can create a new scarf. Make a stunning blanket by adding the double crochet stitch to your repertoire.

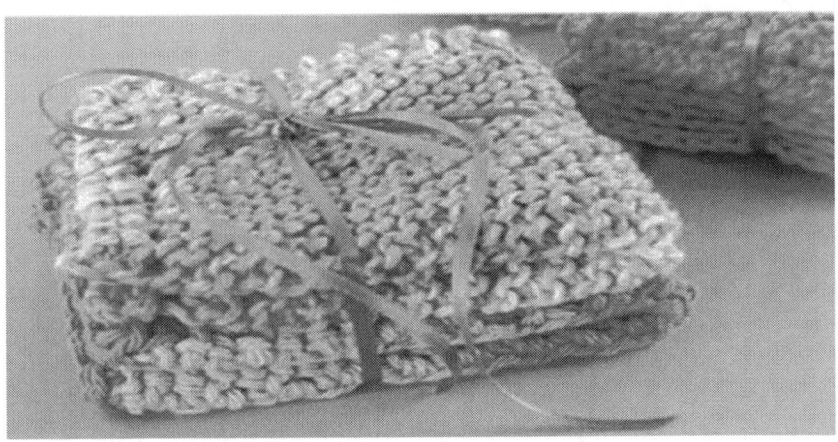

It's important to know, however, that there's a slight learning curve when you're starting out. Any new skill would fit into that category. The phrase "practice makes perfect" applies here. Put a lot of practice into it and be patient with yourself. Creating fun things such as scarves and hats is a great way to practice.

RELIEVES STRESS

It's a known fact that the mind and body are interconnected. On a physical and emotional level. "Mind over matter" is a phrase you've heard before, but why bring it up now? Because *there is a connection between stress and health.*

When you're stressed, you usually know and feel it. You can feel it in your bones, your skin, your hair, and even in your muscles. The change and improvement you see in your physical condition will happen as you relieve that stress, bit by bit. There will be a difference, but it may take time.

MENTAL STAMINA IS IMPROVED BY CROCHETING

In multiple studies, crochet has been proven to improve mental stamina and stave off Alzheimer's and dementia by altering brain chemistry. Several studies have found that crocheting can reduce dementia symptoms by 50 percent according to research conducted by Dr. Yonas Geda, MD, at the Mayo Clinic. That's incredible!

People of all ages can benefit from crocheting's cognitive benefits, which extend beyond Alzheimer's and dementia. In the mail tomorrow, I'm most likely to receive a crochet gift basket if I tell you how often I forget where I put my phone. The number of studies that have found that crocheting and knitting can decrease the risk of dementia by between 30 and 50 percent is astounding! Studies show that crocheting improves cognitive performance overall as a result of sustained focus and concentration.

You're actually making so much more than a scarf or hat. Besides sharpening your brain, decreasing depression and anxiety, distracting from chronic pain, and slowing the onset of dementia, research also shows that it's effective at sharpening your brain. Researchers even suggest people who participate in hobbies like crochet have healthier brains and memories compared to those who do not. In order to build and maintain neural pathways in the brain, sensory stimulation appears to be crucial.

IT HELPS WITH PAIN MANAGEMENT

The process of crocheting requires concentration and focus, as previously mentioned. Several studies have shown that crocheting or knitting is beneficial in reducing pain because you are focusing on something other than your discomfort. During your crochet session, you should be able to lessen your discomfort by concentrating on your abilities.

IT IMPROVES MEMORY

A previously mentioned benefit of crocheting is that it improves cognitive abilities. A remarkable way in which it manifests itself is through the enhancement of memory. The stitching and design of crochet are dependent on your memory to complete a design. Changing colors or moving to the next row or round requires you to keep track of your progress. It is very beneficial to repeat the action in this regard. Practice makes perfect, and the more you practice, the better your memory will become.

IMPROVES YOUR MINDSET

The more you create, the more focused you become. You're better at problem-solving, and you're able to break through emotional walls more effectively. For this reason, it is beneficial for people to create during times of stress, grief, sadness, joy, excitement, and anger. As a result, in doing so you will be able to experience deeper healing and gratitude. That's awesome for your mindset growth! Managing emotions becomes easier when you're able to think and feel them on a deeper level. You're more willing to ask for help when you need it. When it comes to helping their patients open up, therapy counselors often suggest a creative outlet like crafting.

INCREASES HAPPINESS

You've probably heard of flow — it's the state you get in when you're completely absorbed in something. When working on a project, have you ever completely lost track of time and self? There you have it. That's flow. Your heart rate is slowed, your anxiety is reduced, and your mood is boosted.

Flow isn't the only factor that contributes to your happiness. A repetitive creative motion like crocheting, drawing, or writing facilitates flow, and all these tasks produce results. The moment you produce a result, no matter what it is, your brain is flooded with dopamine, that feel-good chemical that motivates you to succeed. Whether or not you're aware of your increased happiness, the hit of dopamine you get after being in flow will drive and influence you toward similar behavior.

CROCHET IS RELAXING

The benefits of crocheting go beyond coping with anxiety and depression. It also relieves tension and promotes relaxation. You can relax with crochet's rhythmic movements and let the yarn flow over your crochet hook to distract you from your problems. Relaxation releases feel-good chemicals like serotonin in the body. Reducing blood pressure and heart rate is one of the health benefits of serotonin production.

When your two-year-old is awake, crocheting is far less stressful to do, especially since there are no needles or thin threads to get tangled up in. Worst case scenario, you'll have to worry about them jabbing their sibling with the hook or unraveling your yarn. Isn't it irritating? Yes. But, is it easier to clean? Yes, as well.

Similar to meditation, crocheting promotes relaxation. Relaxation reduces anxiety and depression symptoms by putting you in a very peaceful, relaxed state. Serotonin, a neurotransmitter that produces feel-good thoughts and feelings, is produced in our brains when we crochet. Cortisol is another stress hormone that is lowered by it. The act of crocheting allows me to feel more relaxed when I'm anxious or upset. An achievement and feeling of well-being are always present when I complete a project.

CROCHET THROUGH INSOMNIA

Sleep deprivation is a terrible experience. Sleep is much more difficult if you're exhausted yet unable to sleep, so you're frustrated. Fortunately, yarn crafting can save the day! Your body and mind will often become relaxed enough for sleep if you concentrate on a gentle, calming, easy, repetitive crochet or knitting craft. As reported by Stitchlinks, an organization based in the UK that conducts research into knitting's benefits, a study conducted by Professor Herbert Benson of Mind/Body

Medical Institute found that 100% of insomnia patients improved their sleep as a result of knitting and crocheting, with 90% able to stop taking their medication.

CROCHETING HELPS WITH MOVEMENT AND DEXTERITY

The benefits extend to arthritis sufferers as well. The movements of crochet contribute to mobility. Special hooks for arthritic hands are also available. Having arthritis or limited hand and finger motion might also benefit you from crocheting. Crocheting's repeated action preserves or increases flexibility in your fingers and hands, and there are many hooks available to alleviate any discomfort caused by prolonged crochet time.

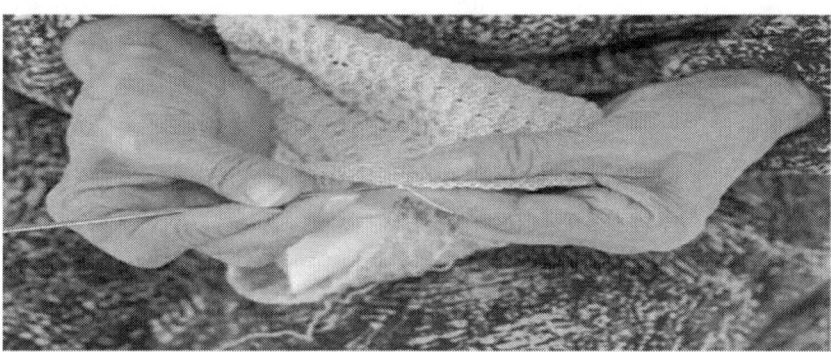

Several small yet precise movements are involved in crocheting. Over time, we become more fluid in the movements of our hands and fingers as we gain expertise. As well as keeping finger joints supple, those repeated movements develop hand muscles and wrist muscles.

IT LOWERS YOUR HEART RATE AND BLOOD PRESSURE

Several health benefits are associated with crocheting. There's no denying that it's a lot of fun. A lower blood pressure and pulse rate, for example, can result from lovely crocheted yarn art.

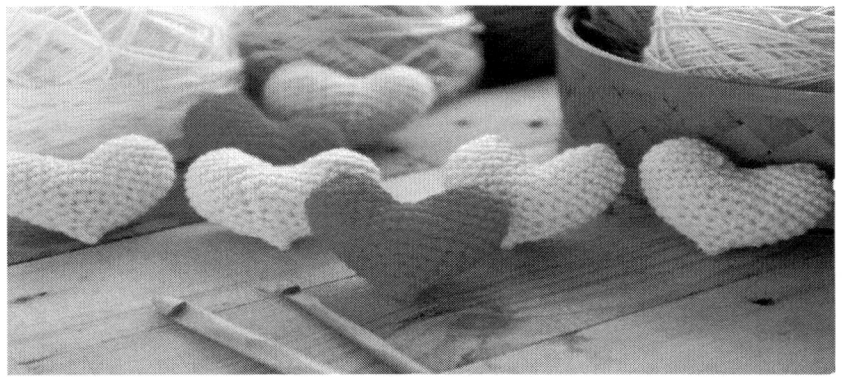

Each one of us faces a variety of pressures in our daily lives. Cortisol, a stress hormone, is released when you are stressed. An array of symptoms and disorders can result from high cortisol levels. Conversely, crocheting lowers cortisol levels.

IT IMPROVES MATH SKILLS AND FINE MOTOR SKILLS

Crocheting will improve your math skills, whether you believe it or not. Yes, that is correct. This is due to the fact that crocheting requires counting. You add, multiply, divide, and measure. I feel that counting helps me to relax. It eventually falls unconscious. You just do it without giving it any thought. However, while you do it, you are developing and enhancing your arithmetic abilities and creating neural connections in your brain. Crochet's repeated action also helps to improve your fine motor skills and hand-eye coordination.

The more you create, the more focused you become. You're better at problem-solving, and you're able to break through emotional walls more effectively. For this reason, it is beneficial for people to create during times of stress, grief, sadness, joy, excitement, and anger. As a result, in doing so you will be able to experience deeper healing and gratitude. That's awesome for your mindset growth!

Managing emotions becomes easier when you're able to think and feel them on a deeper level. You're more willing to ask for help when you need it. When it comes to helping their patients open up, therapy counselors often suggest a creative outlet like crafting.

IT PREVENTS MINDLESS EATING

My habit of nibbling at night usually coincides with watching television. Eating is an aimless process for me. The movie snacking is another story altogether. There is always a feeling that I need something to eat when it's movie time, regardless of whether or not I am hungry. The problem of mindless snacking is also prevalent.

Consequently, I crochet while watching TV at night as a way to relieve stress. If I am occupied with something besides chips, I won't reach for them. Creative thinking changes the brain. Those of you who love data and statistics will be interested in knowing that creative activities (like yarn art) can actually change your brain for the better and relieve stress.

8

THE SECRET TO A 20-MINUTE SOLUTION

Whenever you make a simple double scarf, take a moment to consider how you feel. The thoughts that run through your head might be completely unrelated to what you are doing. Imagine doing it intentionally when you are facing a situation or problem that requires a solution. Do not overthink and worry about this project's outcome. Instead, get out your hook, yarn, and a simple project.

You might be surprised at how many ways you can come up with to solve that problem or situation after crafting for about 20 minutes. Get a pen and paper and jot down all the ideas that come to mind. A list of your priorities is easy when you craft because you can think outside the box when you do it. When preparing for a trip, I use this to remember everything I need to pack. This "forced meditation" can be used to help with any issue that needs attention - about 20 minutes of simple craft work should suffice.

9

CROCHET ENCOURAGES SOCIAL CONNECTION BY COMBATING LONELINESS

The fact that crochet brings people together is one of the reasons you can envision your grandmother and her friends sitting on the porch with their crafts projects and gossiping together. Individuals can interact in a variety of ways when crocheting, both virtually and in person. With the advent of social media platforms such as Instagram, crochet has become a craze among our generation, and crafters can show off their products and receive feedback from their followers. Creating a crochet club can also be a great way to meet new people!

There is even a social network dedicated to yarn artists. The knitting and crocheting community at Ravelry shares patterns, to-do lists, and triumphant images of completed projects. The crochet community is a huge one, and despite the fact that I crochet on my own, I share a lot of passions with others enthusiasts. It would be great if you could find someone to crochet with. You don't even need to be in the same room as your buddy to enjoy some time together.

CROCHET ENCOURAGES SOCIAL CONNECTION BY COMBATING LONELINESS

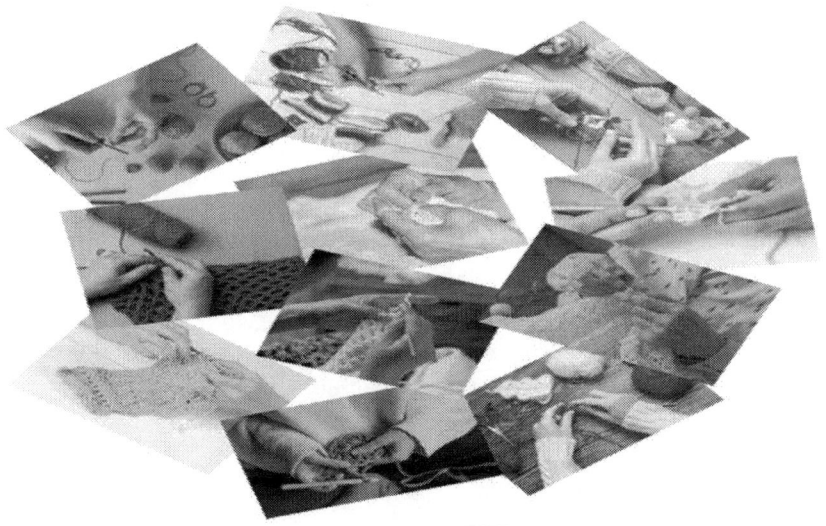

It is possible to participate free of charge in several internet forums. There is a Facebook page where individuals can communicate, discuss ideas, and ask for help or items. The Pinterest website is another great resource for finding yarn ideas and meeting others. The more people you engage with who are interested in your hobby, the less lonely you will feel. It's true that we have all felt increasingly isolated recently because of the epidemic. It is therefore possible to feel less alone by joining online communities like these.

In addition to boosting, one's self-esteem, crocheting boosts one's creativity. The feeling of accomplishment I get after completing a nice project is very satisfying for me. In addition to sharing photos of my projects, selling them is one of my biggest joys.

HEALTH BENEFITS OF CROCHETING

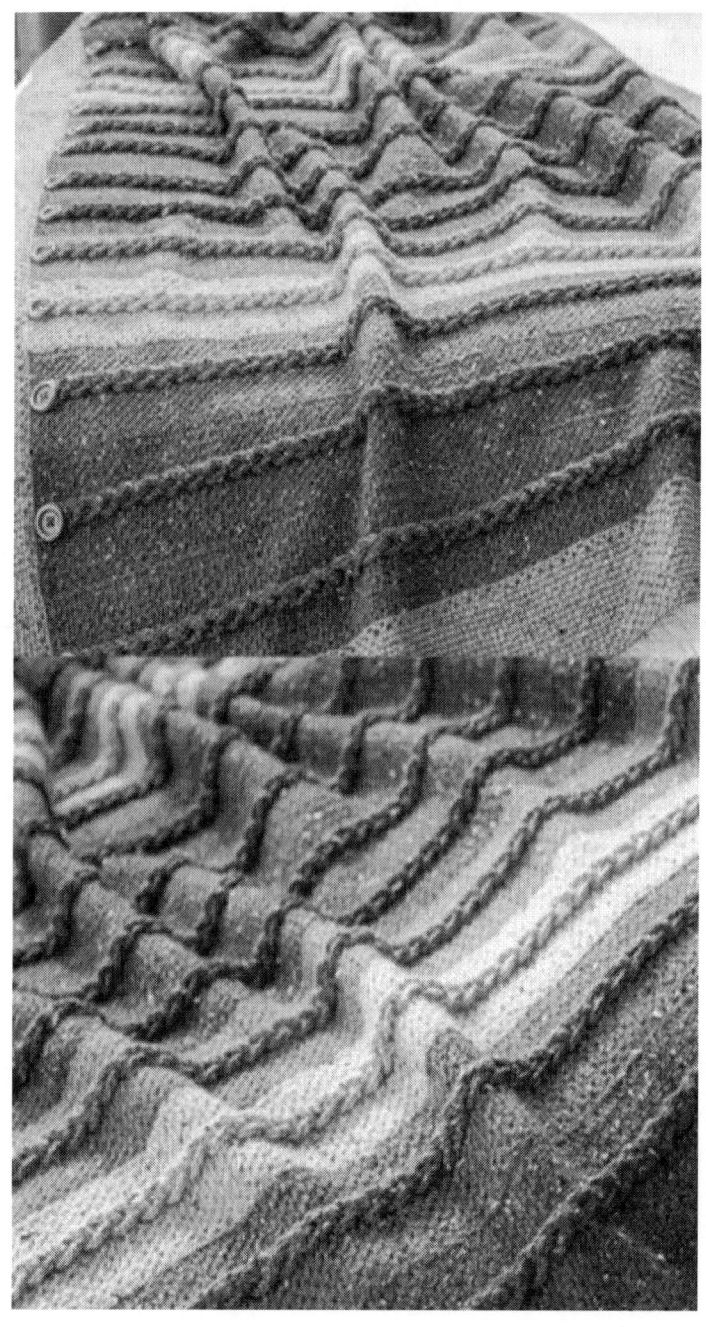

CROCHET ENCOURAGES SOCIAL CONNECTION BY COMBATING LONELINESS

Making mistakes doesn't bother me much except for a brief moment of frustration. It is easy to reverse the mistake that you made when crocheting so that you can start over whenever you make one. It often takes me a while to realize I have made a mistake after I have completed the task. It is inevitable. Ultimately, we are all just humans. My dog usually receives it in those situations. A large part of his toy collection is comprised of misshapen baby booties. Our satisfaction is therefore mutual.

10

CROCHET PROVIDES ENDLESS GIFT POSSIBILITIES!

Creating attractive wearable art is the main reason for learning to crochet. The items I enjoy crocheting most are those for newborns and children. In addition to being quick and easy to make, they allow you to use your imagination to great effect. The most important thing to remember about crochet is that it isn't just used for making cute baby hats. In addition to making items for children, you can also make some items for adults. The creation of scarves and wraps, for example, is simple and ideal for sewers just starting out. Another enjoyable and simple DIY is making a wine gift bag.

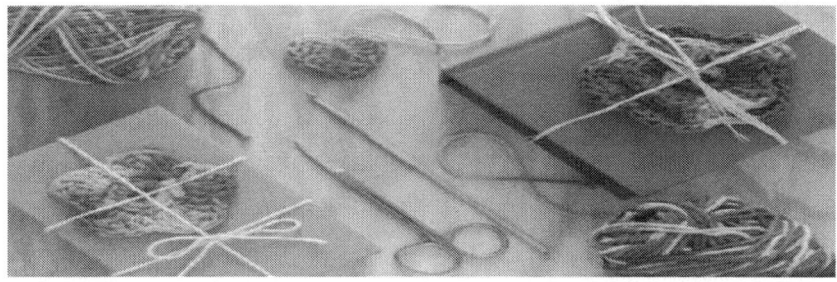

CROCHET PROVIDES ENDLESS GIFT POSSIBILITIES!

Making unique, handcrafted gifts for family and friends is possible when you learn how to crochet. It is said that it is better to give than to receive. The Friends characters (complete with Phoebe and her guitar) are a popular theme for crochet amigurumi figures right now.

The majority of the afghans and shawls I have given away over the years are granny stripe afghans, along with scarves, necklaces, and plush animals. Whether you're looking for doilies, baby blankets, or cardigans, there are many gift options available! Store-bought presents cannot compare to homemade ones. Creating crocheted gifts for family and friends is one of my favorite things to do. Personalization makes it much more meaningful. In a sense, I'm giving them a piece of myself. As well as personalizing the goods for each person, I can make them to order.

11

CROCHET HAS INCOME-EARNING POTENTIAL

Yes, it is right. I crochet because **I LOVE** doing it. But I don't mind that I may sell a large portion of what I create. Purchasing yarn will be the only real cost once you get started. It is nearly impossible to lose money when you sell your creations. Beyond clothing, crochet home decor items like pillows, wall hangings, rugs, and throws are easy to make and look great in any home. Then there's Amigurumi – crochet stuffed dolls and toys.

Crochet has already been discussed for its numerous health benefits. But, what if I told you that crocheting may also help you save money and can result in a lucrative side hustle if those reasons are not already enough to entice you to start crocheting now? The possibilities really are endless!

CROCHET HAS INCOME-EARNING POTENTIAL

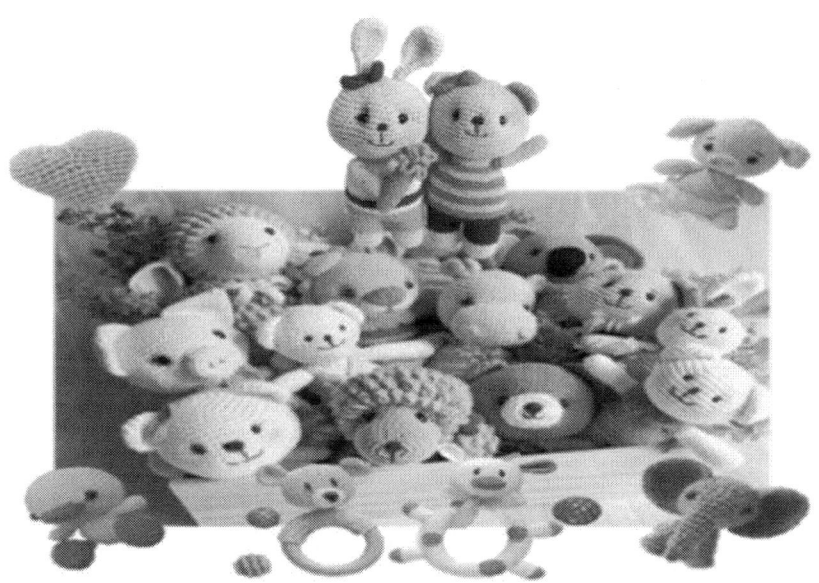

You don't have to start crocheting with the intention of one day opening an Etsy shop, but if you love it and improve your skills, you could eventually sell your work. Considering it will allow you to showcase your hard work in the future, it's a good idea! Consider starting your own internet business or looking for local craft events in your area. Don't let anyone tell you that imparting your knowledge and talent is wrong (and earning an extra income in the process).

Etsy has a section dedicated to crochet products. There are also yarn, supplies, and designs you can buy there, in addition to selling items. In addition to getting ideas for new projects, I also use them as a resource. Selling your products online is possible also on other platforms, such as Shopify.

It's my hope that you and your children are persuaded that crocheting could be a fun new activity. If my godchildren were interested, I would teach them to crochet. (Last summer, I taught my best friend's children to crochet.)

12

DONATIONS CAN BE MADE TO HOSPITALS OR TO THOSE IN NEED

It is possible to sell your finished artwork in addition to donating it to hospitals or homeless shelters. The simple and quick nature of infant hats makes me make them a lot. It doesn't hurt that they're always so adorable. Having the opportunity to sell them is enjoyable. I feel even better when I give them away. As a result, once a month I donate what I have to a hospital for newborns in the neighborhood.

DONATIONS CAN BE MADE TO HOSPITALS OR TO THOSE IN NEED

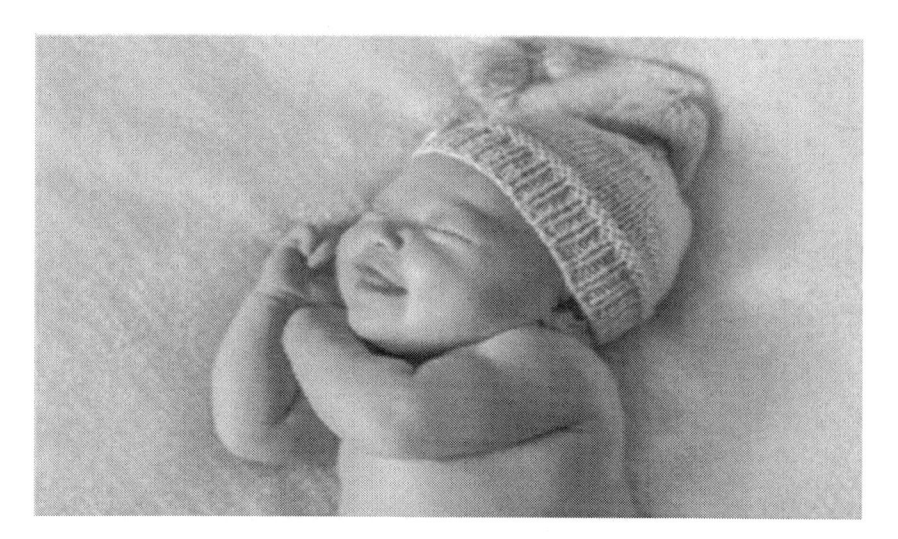

Furthermore, I crochet adult caps and socks to donate to drug rehabilitation centers and homeless shelters. They always appreciate the new clothes, and I like assisting others. It's what I call a win-win situation.

13

15 AWESOME RESOURCES FOR BEGINNERS

If you're sold and ready to get started, check out these 15 awesome resources for beginners to learn how to crochet:
BEST CROCHET BOOKS FOR BEGINNERS:
1. **How To Crochet: A Complete Guide for Absolute Beginners By Alison McNicol.**

As someone who has never crocheted be, this book was written for the novice of crochet beginners. As the author walks beginners through the crocheting process one step at a time, she covers hooks, yarns, and proper holding techniques before moving on to stitches. In addition to the full-color illustrations of stitches and beginner projects, this book has excellent directions.

2. **Crochet Techniques & Tips By Publications International Ltd.**

In this book on learning to crochet, step-by-step photos demonstrate each stitch and technique in detail, making it very easy to follow. This book doesn't contain any beginner projects, but if you want the basics, it's an excellent investment. Despite its small size and low price, it is very practical and useful.

3. **Literary Yarns: Crochet Projects Inspired By Classic Books**

By Cindy Wang.

This crochet project book is perfect if you constantly make literary references only a few people can understand. Creating characters from classic novels requires just a basic knowledge of crochet stitches. As an Anne of Green Gables fan, this one is definitely on my list.

4. Complete Crochet Course: The Ultimate Reference Guide By Shannon And Jason Mullet-Bowlsby.

This reference guide is the only one you'll ever need for learning how to crochet. The Complete Crochet Course includes ten beginner patterns in addition to all the basics.

5. The Chicks With Sticks Guide To Crochet: Learn To Crochet With More Than 30 Cool, Easy Patterns By Nancy Queen And Mary Ellen O'Connell.

Whether you're a total beginner or an experienced crocheter, this witty beginner's crochet guide has a range of techniques and patterns for you to choose from. There are 30 stylish and fashion-forward projects included for a variety of tastes and skill levels. According to the authors, you can learn how to crochet in less time than it takes to potty train a stubborn toddler (ok, so I added that part).

BEST YOUTUBE INSTRUCTIONAL VIDEOS:

My favorite thing about instructional videos is that I can rewind and stop as many times as needed to master a concept. What's up with my godchildren not knowing what "rewind" means?!) All of the creators I'm about to introduce you have been working in crochet for quite some time, and they're all known for their ease of use when it comes to helping others learn the art.

6. How To Crochet For Absolute Beginners Playlist From Bella Coco

Almost 960,000 people are subscribers to Bella Coco's YouTube channel because Sarah-Jayne Fragola knows how to work a hook. Whether you're a visual learner or a more kinesthetic learner, Bella

Coco's playlist for absolute beginners can provide a solid foundation before you investigate her other tutorials and projects. The videos are each under ten minutes long, so replaying them for better understanding isn't terribly time-consuming.

7. How To Crochet For Beginners From The Crochet Crowd

Both the Crochet Crowd's YouTube channel and their website offer incredibly simple-to-follow videos and tutorials. Starting with the basics and moving through common stitches, this video covers crochet from beginning to end.

8. Learn To Crochet Playlist From Moogly Blog

Tamara Kelly at Moogly Blog provides another set of excellent beginner crochet videos. Most of the videos in the playlist are only about two minutes long, so I like that each covers a specific stitch or skill. Organizing them this way allows you to quickly find what you require without having to sort through long video content.

9. How To Crochet For Beginners - Left-Hand Part 1 Tutorial From Naztazia

The world is made for righties, as I know from firsthand experience that my goddaughter Lilly is the only left-handed person on either side of our family. Most beginner crochet videos assume that viewers are right-handed, making it very difficult for lefties to learn how to crochet. Those differences shouldn't stop lefties from using them, but there are some differences to acknowledge. Lefty crochet basics are thoroughly covered by Donna Wolfe from Naztazia, including different stitches and finishing techniques.

10. How To Crochet – Very Slow Demonstration From Kristin's Crochet Tutorials

You don't need to feel ashamed if you need to slow things down based on the millions of views this video has received. Even if you have to pause and rewind this tutorial several times (like I did), you will know exactly what to do each step of the way as you watch the extra-slow demonstration of how to get started with single crochet stitches, and then you can work up to regular speed tutorials from there.

BEST ONLINE RESOURCES:

You should never underestimate the importance of bookmarking several websites or blogs, in addition to books and videos. In addition to free tutorials, you can also find gorgeous crochet patterns and additional assistance (often free) on these sites.

11. Craftyminx: Crochet School

A great feature of this particular blog is the official Crochet School course that the blogger has created, complete with a syllabus. Dana is on hand to assist you at any time while you work through the modules, and it is all completely free of charge. As you progress through the course, she may address these questions in subsequent modules.

12. Crochet Guru: Crochet Made Simple

Its layout is so user-friendly that I am a huge fan of Crochet Guru's website. The following are some free tutorials that Bobbie Thomson has created for beginner crocheters (all of which are available online). Each tutorial has been made into left-handed crochet videos along with pictures. Bobbie, you're doing a wonderful job fighting for crochet equity.

13. Mama In A Stitch

Visiting Mama in a Stitch's website makes you feel like you're reconnecting with your inner crochet Zen. You can receive crochet tips and additional resources by subscribing to owner Jessica's mailing list. This is one of the best sites for free crochet patterns. If you like what you see, you can sign up to be a Mamas Maker Member for a small annual fee.

14. Cherry Heart Blog

For all the podcast listeners out there, here's one for you. You'll find endlessly engaging content at Sandra's Cherry Heart Blog, from her podcast to an incredibly detailed stitch directory, whether you are just getting started with crochet or have been doing it for a while. Besides dividing crochet techniques by skill level, she also provides advanced tutorials once you master the beginner stitch.

15. Melanie Ham

As part of Melanie's holistic DIY approach, she offers crochet, quilting, and sewing resources. The Beginner Crochet Guide includes videos and instructions for newbies on how to crochet. Melanie recently created this guide for beginners. You can access all of the videos on the guide page, and you can also purchase premium crochet courses depending on what you'd like to accomplish.

14

CONCLUSION

IT ALL COMES DOWN TO THIS
When your mind is being taken care of in a more positive way, your body will follow. Creating is one way to encourage a healthy mind and move toward happiness and less stress. Changing the way you speak to yourself is another. Celebrate what you did right. You believe the stories you tell yourself. When you accomplish a project, make sure you celebrate that win! Don't go through looking for mistakes, take a good look at what you did right. That small change will add up every time and your mind will start to believe in your progress and will reward you for that!

HOW TO MAKE CHANGE HAPPEN
Embrace a new way of thinking. You can welcome a more positive viewpoint when you focus on improving your way of thinking. A healthy lifestyle could result from spending time with loved ones, spending more time outside, eating healthier meals, and getting outdoors more often. Choosing life choices that will help you thrive and live the life you deserve. Mental health disorders such as depression, anxiety, and stress can be treated with a healthier lifestyle.

It is obvious that there are several compelling reasons to learn how to crochet now. It's a healthy and enjoyable activity. You can pick up a simple crochet project next time you're feeling stressed or emotionally depleted. Take a look at what happens when you let go and let the craft guide your thoughts. It might surprise you how quickly your physical tension begins to disappear. The feeling of calmness should also start to return to you. You can even make some money doing it. Furthermore, it enables you to create one-of-a-kind wearable art that you can keep or give away.

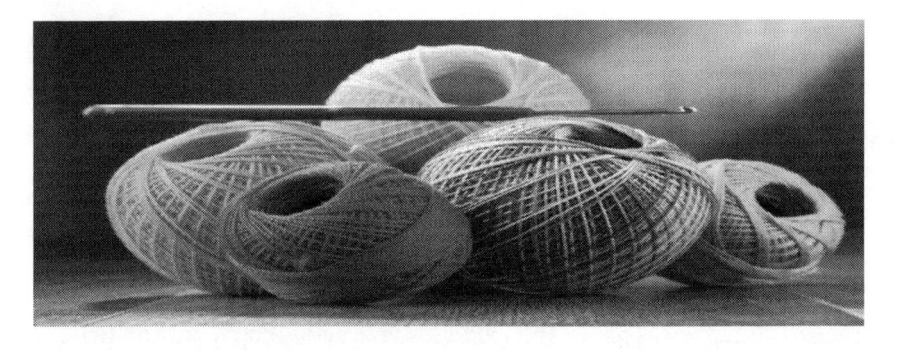

I really hope you enjoyed reading this book as much as I enjoyed writing it! What are you waiting for now? Gather your yarn and get ready to hook!

It would be greatly appreciated if you could leave a positive review on Amazon if you found this book useful.

15

RESOURCES

Crowd, T. C. (2019, March 8). *10 Great Reasons to Crochet | BEGINNER | The Crochet Crowd.* YouTube. Retrieved September 6, 2022, from https://www.youtube.com/watch?v=F8Cnto2yM9c&feature=youtu.be

D, M. (2021, March 25). *Top 15 Reasons Why You Should Take up Crochet Today.* REASONS TO SKIP THE HOUSEWORK. Retrieved September 6, 2022, from https://www.reasonstoskipthehousework.com/take-up-crochet/

Jess. (2019, June 28). *Reasons to Do Crochet | Superprof.* We Love Prof - Superprof Blog. Retrieved September 6, 2022, from https://www.supeprof.com/blog/why-crochet/

Lion Brand Yarn. (2021, August 7). *Mayo Clinic Reports That Knitting May Reduce Alzheimer's Risk by 30-50%.* Lion Brand Notebook. Retrieved September 6, 2022, from https://blog.lionbrand.com/mayo-clinic-reports-that-knitting-may-reduce-alzheimers-risk-by-30-50/

Polino, M. B. (n.d.). *Crochet Therapy.* THE ASSOCIATION FOR CREATIVITY IN COUNSELING. Retrieved September 6, 2022, from https://www.counseling.org/docs/default-source/aca-acc-creative-activities-clearinghouse/crochet-therapy.pdf?sfvrsn=6#:~:text=Crafting%

20May%20Reduce%20or%20Postpone,already%20experiencing%20signs%20of%20dementia.

Simplydaisy. (2015, March 16). How to Crochet for Absolute Beginners: Part 1. YouTube. Retrieved September 6, 2022, from https://www.youtube.com/watch?v=aAxGTnVNJiE&feature=youtu.be

Stahl, A. (2018, July 25). *Here's How Creativity Actually Improves Your Health*. Forbes. Retrieved September 6, 2022, from https://www.forbes.com/sites/ashleystahl/2018/07/25/heres-how-creativity-actually-improves-your-health/?sh=27e4464713a6

The Knotted Nest. (2021, February 13). *Why crochet is making a comeback (and why you should be part of it!): Modern crochet for the home and family*. The Knotted Nest. Retrieved September 6, 2022, from https://knottednest.com/why-crochet-is-making-a-comeback-and-why-you-should-be-part-of-it/

Woodbury, A. (2022, June 16). *Solve Your Stress Problems in 20 Minutes*. Happily Hooked Crochet Magazine. Retrieved September 6, 2022, from https://www.happilyhooked.com/blog/solve-stress-problems/

Ziegmont, T. (2021a, May 31). *15 Best Resources for Learning to Crochet*. Feels Like Home. Retrieved September 6, 2022, from https://feelslikehomeblog.com/best-resources-for-learning-to-crochet/

Ziegmont, T. (2021b, October 28). *12 Reasons Why Crocheting Should Be Your New Hobby*. Feels Like Home™. Retrieved September 6, 2022, from https://feelslikehomeblog.com/12-reasons-why-crocheting-should-be-your-new-hobby/#:%7E:text=Not%20only%20does%20crochet%20act,yarn%20over%20your%20crochet%20hook.

Made in the USA
Columbia, SC
19 September 2022